seduce

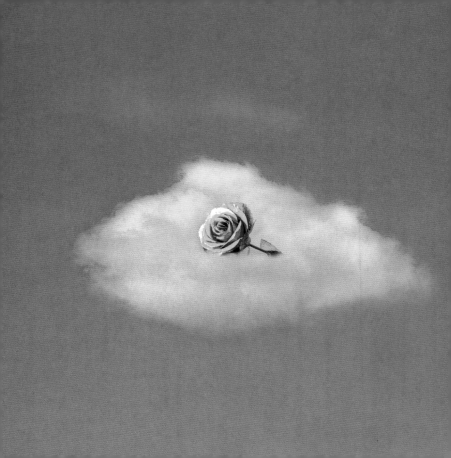

seduce

100 tips to arouse

Eva Gizowska

BARRON'S

First edition for North America published in
2003 by Barron's Educational Series, Inc.

Copyright © **MQ Publications Ltd** 2003

All rights reserved. No part of this book
may be reproduced in any form, by
photostat, microfilm, xerography, or any
others means, or incorporated into any
information retrieval system, electronic or
mechanical, without the written permission
of the copyright owner.

All inquiries should be addressed to:
Barron's Educational Series, Inc.
250 Wireless Boulevard
Hauppauge, NY 11788
http://www.barronseduc.com

International Standard Book
No. 0-7641-5698-5

Library of Congress Catalog Card No.
2003101024

SERIES EDITOR: **Yvonne Deutch**
DESIGN: **Balley Design Associates**

Printed in China
9 8 7 6 5 4 3 2 1

contents

introduction

You don't have to be good looking to be sexually alluring.
That's because seduction has very little to do with physical
perfection, and everything to do with the way you act.
Being seductive can be a million different things. It may be
the special way you look, touch, and talk that signals your
subliminal intentions. You can also create an arousing
environment with color, music, and sound. Seduction is
what adds excitement to a romance and keeps a steady
relationship fresh.

Fortunately, there are many ways in which you can make
yourself more seductive to your partner and *SEDUCE*
offers you a revealing insight into 100 of these crucial

secrets. So, if you're looking for new and exciting ways to enhance your love life, attract a new lover, or just make yourself more appealing to the opposite sex, this is where *SEDUCE* can help.

Here you'll find 100 enlightening tips on how to be more alluring. These include ways to entice and arouse with touch, taste, and scent, and also with your mental attitude. Most of all, always remember that being seductive is about being humorous, loving, and warm, not coolly manipulative. So, try some of these intriguing tips and see how easy it is to add a spicy, sensuous ingredient to your love life, and an extra sparkle to your eyes.

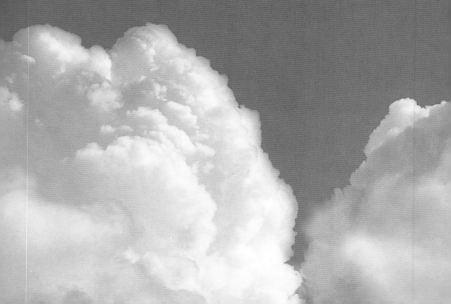

CHAPTER ONE

seductive touch

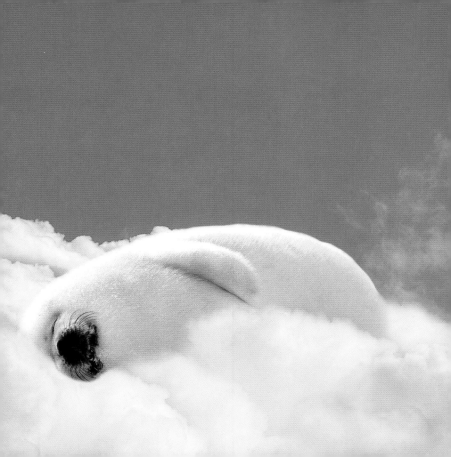

1 Head for love

Your lover will feel blissful after this relaxing head massage. Using your fingertips, start at the temples and apply pressure in firm, circular motions. Work upward, toward the center of the head, around the sides, and down toward the base of the neck. For an ultra-relaxing effect, focus on the center of the head (you should feel a slight indent there) and the four points around it. Use your thumb on these points, and massage in an anti-clockwise direction (for women) or clockwise (for men) for 15 seconds each way. Finish the head massage by gently pulling at the hair roots all over the head.

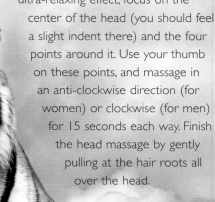

2 Strokes for folks

At the end of a tiring day, you and your lover may want to get relaxed and intimate with a sensual stroking session. But, first set the scene. Choose a quiet, comfortable place such as the bedroom, dim the lights, and put on some soothing music. Don't worry, you don't have to be a trained massage expert. Just go with the flow, and do what feels natural, starting with some gentle touching and stroking. Then, get your partner to lie on his or her stomach, while you kneel on one side. Rub your hands to warm them. Now, place each hand flat at the base of the spine, and lightly work your way upward. Knead, stroke, or glide (whichever feels best) your way up along the back and across the shoulders and neck (working toward the heart). Be creative and experiment by using different kinds of pressure and strokes.

3 Sexy scents

A massage with deliciously scented oils can make your lover dizzy with pleasure. Ask your partner to sniff, then choose his or her favorites from a selection of oils renowned for their powerful aphrodisiac qualities: try florals such as jasmine, rose, neroli, ylang-ylang, as well as clary sage, sandalwood, and frankincense. Make up your customized blend by using five to six drops (of one or more oils) diluted in a carrier oil such as sweet almond, jojoba, or grapeseed. Warm the oil in your hands before applying.

4 Soothing touch

Stress is a guaranteed passion killer. Here's a simple, tender way to help your lover unwind after a tense day. Get your partner to lie down comfortably on his or her back, head comfortably on your knees. Using your thumbs, gently massage the points between the eyebrows. After a minute or so, slowly glide your thumbs toward the temples. Massage in small circular movements as you do so. Next, place your fingertips on the lower jaw—in front of the ears and under the cheekbones—and gently massage the area. This helps reduce muscular tension. Move downward, and massage chin and neck with light, gentle strokes.

5 Sexy sparklers

If your relationship is getting a tad predictable, here are a few tips on how to pep things up. Together with your partner, create a wish list of your favorite little love treats—these may include smoochie dancing together, reading a poem, sending a soppy e-mail, whispering sweet nothings on the phone, or simply feeding each other chocolate. Then, delight your lover with a surprise sprinkling of daily, mini-seductions. They take just a few minutes each—but make sure at least three involve physical touch. Fleeting touches like these will ignite the sexual spark.

6 Sensational

Pleasure your darling with the fleeting touch of different textures on the skin. Fabrics such as silk and velvet can feel gorgeously sensual—for instance, take a delicate silk scarf, slide it delicately along your partner's naked body, and enjoy the thrilled reaction. Or, take a baby-soft feather—ostrich is perfect—and, while your lover's eyes are closed, lightly run it, barely touching, over his or her arms, legs, and back. It's a soothing, swooning, erotic sensation. You'll love it too, so ask your partner to do the same to you. This mutual enjoyment will help you both to explore the many different pleasure points on each other's body.

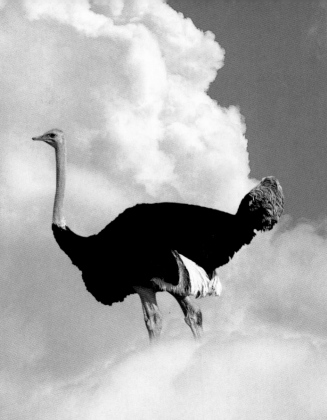

7 Five great kisses

Want to make your kisses more exciting? Then try the following:

- Ice kiss—put an ice cube in your mouth. Take it out when your mouth feels really cold. Now, kiss your partner.
- Eyelid kiss—Watch as your partner's eyes close. Then gently kiss the closed lids.
- Mint kiss—Eat an extra-strong mint, then kiss each other for a supremely invigorating kiss.
- Ear kiss—Whisper a sexy compliment in your lover's ear, and follow up by gently kissing the ear. This will send delicious shivers down the spine.
- Fresh kiss—Brush your teeth together, and when your mouths are still sudsy with paste, kiss.

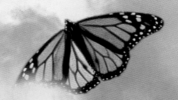

8 Eyelash flutter

Here's a fun way to get close to your loved one. Say "Close your eyes, darling." Then, use your eyelashes like a butterfly, and gently flutter them along the back of the hand, up along the arm, and against the nape of the neck. If you want, you can also flutter your lashes across his or her chest. Finally, gently let your lashes caress your lover's face and cheeks. Slowly and sensuously work your way down to the lips. Then, trace the outline of the lips with your fingers, and give your lover a passionate kiss.

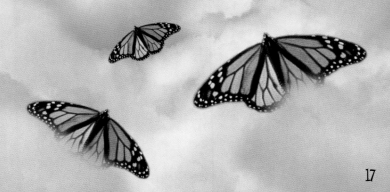

9 Hand in hand

Men rarely look after their hands, so amaze your guy with a sensual hand massage—it's such a loving way to help him unwind and relax, and will also make his hands feel smoother and softer on your body. First, blend a base oil such as jojoba or apricot kernel with a couple of drops of neroli and rose oil. Now massage a few drops into his hand—working on one at a time. Massage the entire hand, using small circular movements, and work the oil in between the finger bones. Then, take

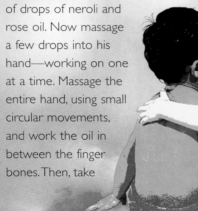

each finger with your opposite hand and massage along the entire length. Use a few more drops for a final massage to both hands—and watch the contented smile appear on his face. With pleasuring like this, he'll be delighted to do the same for you.

10 Kiss hands

Through stroking and touching, you and your lover use your hands to give pleasure to each other. It's easy to forget that the hands are sensitive erotic zones in their own right. Delight your lover by gently taking his or her hand and opening it to reveal the palm. First, stroke the palm with your fingertips, then kiss the center with a long, loving kiss. It's also deliciously sensuous to massage the center of your lover's palm with the tip of your tongue. Finally, take each finger in turn and kiss each tip, one by one.

11 Light up

Lost your love spark? Try these oriental exercises:

- Sit comfortably on the floor with your back straight and legs together. Breathe out and slowly, stretch forward to reach the inside of your ankles. Hold. Return to the starting position.
- Start from the same position as above. Open your legs as wide as possible, keeping your feet flexed. Breathing out, clasp your hands together and reach toward the top of your left foot in one slow stretch. Keep your forehead down. Hold.
- Slowly, return to the start. Repeat with the other foot.

12 Love muscles

Strong pelvic floor muscles are important if a women is to enjoy sex to the utmost. If yours are not as toned as they might be, get yourself back into shape with a simple routine. Known as Kegel exercises, these are designed to pull the pelvic floor muscles inward and upward. You should breathe in as the muscles tighten and breathe out as they relax, and gradually build up a regular daily routine. You'll not only experience stronger, more intense orgasms, your lover will get more pleasure also.

13 Shiatsu

Shiatsu is a Japanese form of massage similar to acupressure. Here are a couple of tips to help boost your libido:

- Place the back of your hands on your back, just below the rib cage. Start to rub the area slowly until you can feel increased warmth. This stimulates your vitality and sexual energy.
- Bend forward slightly and, with your clenched fists, tap from as high up the back as you can reach. Tap all the way down to the buttocks. Focus on the buttocks, until this area feels relaxed. This activates the parasympathetic nervous system, which in turn energizes your sexual organs.

14 Tantric tantalizers

Next time you and you lover feel in a sensual mood, try the following ways to increase your sexual pleasure even further:

- Before you touch each other, rub your hands vigorously. This will increase sensitivity and feeling in your hands.
- Get your partner to sit or stand in a comfortable position and gently "rock" him or her in a swaying, rhythmic manner. Start at the shoulders and move down to the feet.
- Sit, stand, or lie close together—without touching. Close your eyes, breathe deeply, and just enjoy being with each other.

15 Bear hug

Seductive touching doesn't have to be exotic and complicated; one of the sexiest ways to get close and passionate is to snuggle together like friendly bears so that your bodies are in maximum contact. Each of you should lie on your left side, one in front of the other, like "spoons." Whoever is on the outside should cradle the other in his or her arms. Relax and begin synchronizing your breathing, imagining the loving energy of each breath flowing into your lover's body, from the groin to the head. This follows the pathway of energy centers known as chakras.

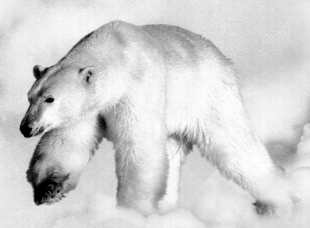

16 Talk and touch

In the early stages of passion, lovers treasure each other's words; but after a while, it's easy to stop communicating so intensely. This can create a distance between you, so you need to make the time to talk. It helps, while you're talking if you touch, hold, and caress each other as a natural part of the conversation.

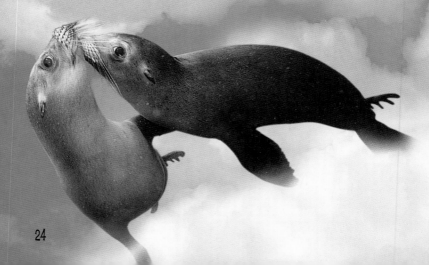

Ideally, you need to set aside some time every day for each other—even if it's only a brief car journey or half an hour before bed. Be straightforward and honest, and really listen to what your partner has to say. Loving attention like this will bring you emotionally closer, and that, in turn, will bring you sexually closer.

17 Get physical

The fitter you are, the better your sex life. According to recent research, when previously sedentary people took up moderate exercise, they reported a 30 percent increase in sexual activity and a 26 percent increase in the number of orgasms they were having. There's a good reason for this. Exercise encourages the production of endorphins, the body's feel-good hormones. So, the more exercise you do, the more positive and energized you will feel. You needn't go to the gym; enjoy dancing with your partner or going for a walk together.

18 Heart to heart

Do this simple, daily Japanese exercise together, facing each other—it will help to keep your hearts open to each other.

- Sit on the floor with your backs straight. Bring your knees up and place the soles of your feet together. Grasp the tops of your feet, and bring them toward your groin.
- Breathe out, open knees, and stretch, bringing your heads toward your feet. Relax, breathe in and repeat.

19 Instant calm

Sex and tension are a bad combination. So, next time one of you is feeling anxious, or stressed, try this simple acupressure technique. You can either do it for yourself or for your partner.

- Using your right thumb, massage the center of your left palm—in oriental medicine, this point is known as the Palace of Anxiety. Massage for a minute or so, until you feel calmer.

20 The inner smile

This delightful Chinese exercise only takes a few minutes—but it does wonders for your mood, gives you a secret inner glow, and boosts your natural sex appeal. Once you've discovered its subtle benefits, you'll want to do it every day.

- Sit in a comfortable place with your back straight.
- Imagine seeing something that will make you smile. Really feel the smile throughout your body.
- Allow the smile to shine out of your eyes.
- Now imagine the smile traveling smoothly and powerfully into all your internal organs.
- Allow the smile to enter your *tan tien* center—this is situated just below your navel.
- Hold this feeling until you are flooded with happiness. Now you can carry on with the day, holding on to the mellow feelings generated by your internal smile. You'll find that your lover will respond warmly to your good vibrations.

CHAPTER TWO

seductive food

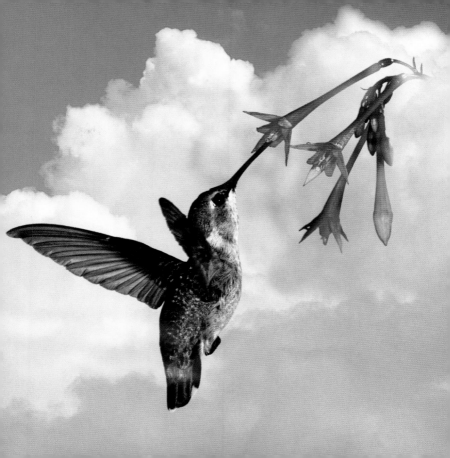

21 What a smoothie

Whip up a spicy love smoothie for your man—it contains vanilla, cardamom, cloves, and cinnamon, delicious aphrodisiac ingredients. You'll need:

1 cup of milk
15 cardamom pods
15 cloves (whole)
2 cinnamon sticks
1 vanilla pod, split
1 small tub vanilla yogurt (frozen)
honey (to taste)

Add cloves, cardamom, cinnamon, and vanilla seeds (from the pod) to the milk. Heat up in a saucepan (but don't boil). Allow to cool, then put in the fridge until chilled. Strain into a blender (minus spices), add the frozen vanilla, yogurt, and honey. Blend into a smoothie and serve.

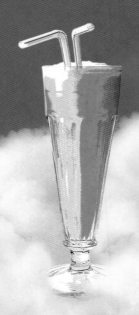

22 Honeymoon heaven

Spice up your love life with a dash of nutmeg and honey added to a cup of hot milk or coffee. Nutmeg was described as a powerful aphrodisiac in Arab, Greek, and Roman writings. In India, it is said that, if you eat a mixture of nutmeg, honey, and half a boiled egg an hour before sex, it will prolong love-making. Honey is also recognized as a well known aphrodisiac. In fact, the term "honeymoon" originated in the days when honey wine (mead) was drunk by the newly wedded couple.

23 Aphrodisiac teas

Yes, certain teas can pep up your sex drive dramatically—here are two of the best:

- Fennel tea: This is available in health stores, in tea bags. The ancient Greeks regarded fennel as a potent sexual stimulant.
- Ginger tea: This ancient spice has been used for centuries to

pep up a low sex drive, as it reputedly increases blood flow to the genitals. Add a few slices of fresh ginger to hot water and let it steep for a few minutes before drinking.

24 Love menu

Certain foods are reputed to have an aphrodisiac effect. This is because they consist of ingredients that help to stimulate desire and increase the libido. For example, bananas contain bromelain, said to enhance male performance. And it's said that the smell of cinnamon has a very arousing effect on men. So get out your cookbook and try this simple love menu:

- Saffron rice and mussels
- Herb salad with basil and pine nuts
- Bananas and strawberries, liberally sprinkled with cinnamon, and drizzled with honey
- Hot chocolate sprinkled with cinnamon

25 Get fruity

For a sensual treat, tempt your lover with some succulent fruits.
Ripe, red strawberries and plump, pink raspberries have long
been regarded as the perfect love fruits—they've been called
"love nipples" in oriental literature. For a sensual feast, dip
strawberries in chocolate. Alternatively, serve wild strawberries
and raspberries with honey or brown sugar and whipped cream.
For a more exotic experience you could try serving
pomegranates. These deep red fruits are recommended in the
Karma Sutra as a way to inflame desire.

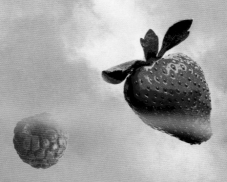

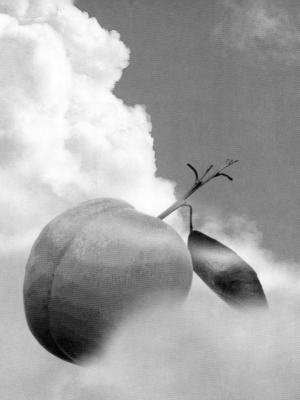

26 Love punch

Mix this aphrodisiac love punch for your lady love—it combines two amazing aphrodisiacs, available in tincture form from health food stores. They are: *damiana,* a Mexican herbal aphrodisiac, and *muira puama,* from Brazil. Mix some fresh orange juice, pineapple juice, and white rum in equal measures. Add a dash of Triple Sec, some lemon juice, 2 vanilla beans, a spoonful of brown sugar, a dash of ground nutmeg, a few drops of *damiana* tincture, and a few drops of *muira puama* tincture. Serve in a pretty glass on a bed of rose petals. Add one kiss.

27 Nuts about you

Pine nuts are rich in zinc, a nutrient that improves male potency and ensures healthy sperm. Zinc is essential for the production of the male sex hormone testosterone. The passion-arousing properties of pine nuts were proclaimed by the Roman poet

Ovid, who listed them as an aphrodisiac in *The Art Of Love*.
Likewise, the physician Galen recommended eating a glass of
thick honey, 20 almonds, and 100 pine nuts before going to bed
(for three consecutive nights) to boost sexual vigor.

28 Wooing with walnuts

Forget peanuts—serve walnuts if you're hoping for romance.
They are packed with essential fatty acids that help to regulate
hormone levels and improve sex drive. In Latin, *juglans*, the word
for walnut, means the glands of Jupiter. This explains why ancient
Romans believed that eating walnuts was good for fertility and
why they scattered walnuts during marriage ceremonies. In
Cleopatra's court, walnuts were stuffed with caramel and served
at weddings. Today, walnuts (and walnut based foods and drinks
such as walnut wines and liqueurs and walnut pâtes) are still
popular aphrodisiacs in parts of Italy and France.

29 Love potion

If you want your next party to go with a swing, serve the following aphrodisiac cocktail:

● Mix peach and mango juices with chilled champagne, in equal measures. Add a dash of lemon juice, stir lightly, and serve. Mangoes are popular aphrodisiacs in India, Mexico, and the Caribbean, while the sensuous-looking peach has been associated with robust sexuality for centuries by the Chinese. Meanwhile, the instant feel-good hit of champagne makes it the perfect drink for seduction, as it promotes a feeling of well-being and also lowers inhibitions.

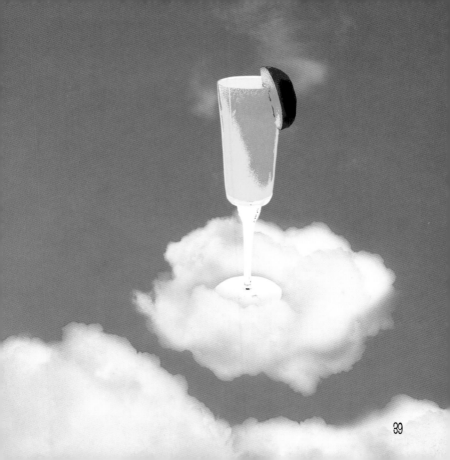

30 Ginseng revival

Tired? Stressed? Libido at floor level? Try a daily dose of ginseng.
There's evidence that it contains compounds with sex hormone
action that might help overcome impotence caused by hormone
deficiency. You can take it as a supplement or as a tea. In Chinese
herbal medicine, ginseng is used to boost energy and vitality,
regulate blood pressure, stimulate the immune system, improve
circulation, and calm the nervous system. It's also an excellent
tonic to help combat the emotional and physical effects of stress.
So, as well as enjoying better sex, life should perk up generally.
For safety, don't take it for longer than one month continuously.

31 Chinese tonic

Sex drive on the wane? Then try a course of Gingko Biloba
supplements. An extract from the Gingko Biloba tree, it is used
as a general tonic in Chinese medicine. It gets the blood flowing

more efficiently through the body, which improves circulation to the extremities. It also increases blood flow to the brain and helps boost mental performance. Enhanced circulation has a stimulating effect and helps to restore our interest in sex.

32 Sex supplements

If your diet is not up to scratch, then you may be short on certain vitamins and minerals that affect your sex life. A low sex drive has been linked to deficiencies in vitamins A, C, E, and B-complex, as well as the minerals zinc and selenium. So, if you're stressed or too busy to eat properly, it might be a good idea to take the following supplements to safeguard your sex life: a daily multivitamin and mineral supplement will fill any nutritional gaps, and you may like to take an extra 500–1000mg Vitamin C. Women may also want to take a daily 500mg capsule of evening primrose oil, which helps to regulate their hormones.

33 Suggestive snack

The ancient Aztec word for the avocado tree was *ahuacuati*, which means "the testicle tree." They thought that this is just what the fruit resembled when it was hanging on the tree. So, avocados—with their delicious flavor and luxuriously fleshy texture—have been thought of as sexy, sensuous, erotic foods ever since. Serve in slices, drizzled with balsamic vinegar, as an aphrodisiac snack. For an extra kick, add a sprinkling of black pepper, which is also considered to be sexually arousing on account of its keen, stimulating effect.

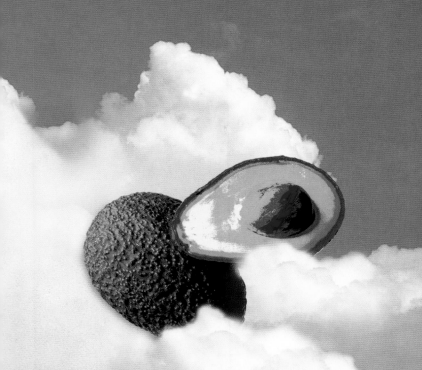

34 Licorice all sorts

Will you become inflamed with desire by chewing on a stick of licorice? Try it and see. Licorice root has been used in Chinese medicine for thousands of years, and is used to induce feelings of lust, in both men and women. It is recommended for women suffering from a low libido, while for men, the smell of licorice is said to increase penile blood flow. Licorice root is available at health food stores—you can also make it into an aphrodisiac tea by mixing a tablespoon of ground licorice root with a tablespoon of fennel seeds. Add boiling water and steep for 20 minutes.

35 Care a fig

Figs were Cleopatra's favorite fruit; so if they hit the spot for her, why not pleasure your lover with fresh figs, served with yogurt or cream and honey. Ever since ancient Egyptian times, these fleshy, succulent fruits—said to resemble a woman's genitalia—

have been considered powerful sexual stimulants. Their reputation is probably based on their visual connotation, as sexual desire is greatly influenced by the mind and imagination. It was certainly considered highly erotic for a man to eat figs in front of a women—in ancient Greece, the arrival of a new fig crop was celebrated by ritual copulation.

36 Seductive seafood

Fishy foods such as oysters, mussels, and caviar are high in minerals such as phosphorus, iodine, and zinc, all vital for maintaining good sexual health. That's why seafood has such a legendary reputation for being a potent aphrodisiac. Oysters have the highest zinc content of all and were popular libido boosters in Roman times. Casanova seems to have believed in them completely—he is said to have maintained his sexual prowess by consuming 50 raw oysters every morning.

37 Hot 'n spicy

Spice up your love life by using sizzling hot chilies in your cooking. They taste great, whether used in a classic chili con carne, or in vegetable or meat dishes. Chilies contain a substance called capsaicin, which has the instant effect of stimulating your circulation. This improved blood flow is said to enhance sexual prowess and performance, especially in men. For that reason, chilies have been used as an aphrodisiac for centuries in South America.

38 Love bundles

It's an ancient phallic symbol of course, and asparagus has been
used as an aphrodisiac for around 3,000 years. In 19th-century
France, bridegrooms ate several servings before their wedding
nights, because of its reputed powers of arousal. Interestingly,
though, we now know that asparagus contains a plant hormone
called asparagocide. It is also packed with selenium, and vitamins
A and C, which are important nutrients for healthy sexual
function. So, go ahead, enjoy feeding your lover succulent spears
dipped in melted butter for a sexy, sensual experience.

39 Sugared almonds

Almonds have been associated with
passion and fertility throughout the ages.
Their aroma is said to be especially arousing
for women. These days, it's still common
practice to hand out little bags of sugared almonds
(as a symbol of fertility) at weddings in Mediterranean countries
such as Spain and Portugal. Serve roasted almonds as a delicious
aphrodisiac snack. Or use them in cake and pastry recipes.

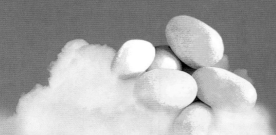

40 Sweets for your sweet

Chocolate means romance? But of course. It contains a powerful natural substance called theobromine, which has an uplifting effect on the mood and boosts energy (in much the same way as caffeine). Chocolate also contains another natural substance, often referred to as the "love drug," because it induces powerful feelings of euphoria, which can be highly addictive. According to scientists, whenever we find someone sexually attractive, levels of this substance are boosted in the brain. Eating chocolate can have a similar effect, and might explain why many people binge on it as a substitute for love.

CHAPTER THREE

seductive scents

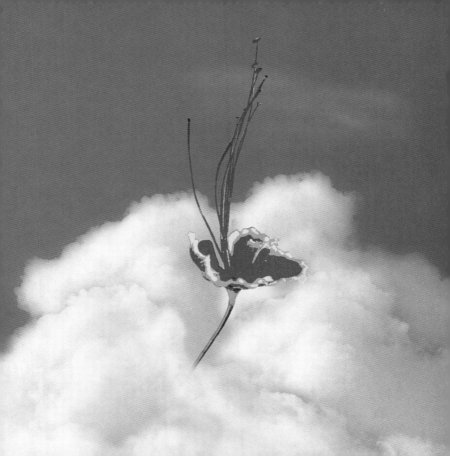

41 A nose for love

You can get your partner in a sensual mood with the intoxicating aroma of essential oils. Use oil burners to suffuse the room with these aphrodisiac scents:

Ylang-ylang This exotic oil will make you both feel euphoric.

Jasmine The aphrodisiac properties of this sweet-scented oil have been known for centuries; it has been used to overcome impotence in men and frigidity in women.

Sandalwood A powerfully aphrodisiac oil that is used in Tantric yoga to awaken sexual energy.

Neroli This has a lingering, sensual aroma that will put you in the mood for love.

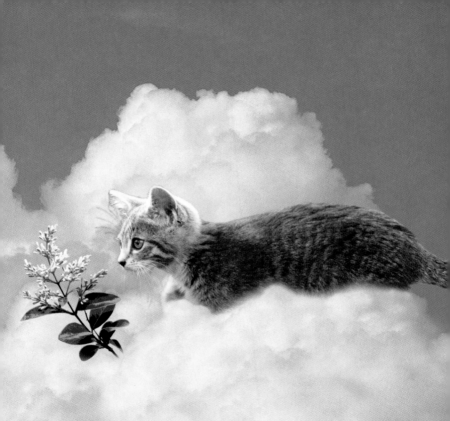

42 Fragrant love charm

If you want to ooze sex appeal and attract a potential partner, try wearing a scented love charm. All you have to do is place a few drops of essential oils such as jasmine, rose, ylang-ylang, or neroli onto a tiny cotton wool ball. Then attach this to a piece of jewelry—for instance, tuck it behind a pendant, or inside a locket. Alternatively, you can apply the oils directly to wooden beads or bracelets. The aphrodisiac aroma of the scented jewelry will secretly and subtly enhance your powers of attraction. It's quite effortless—just smile mysteriously.

43 Vanilla option

Next time you're getting ready for a date, or a romantic evening with your partner, try the effect of a vanilla-scented bath on your desire levels. Simply add a few drops of vanilla essence to the bath, then lie back and let yourself be surrounded by the sweet-scented, aphrodisiac aroma. This can have a subtly arousing effect, which makes you relaxed and more responsive to your lover. Alternatively, you can get your partner in the mood for love with a vanilla-scented bath for two.

44 Heady blend

If you want to make a subliminally erotic impression, create your own aphrodisiac perfume blend, and use it discreetly, but lethally. Choose your favorite scent from jasmine, rose, or ylang-ylang, and combine it with your choice from neroli, orange, lemon, or mandarin oil. Add 8–10 drops to a 30 ml bottle of base oil such as jojoba or sweet almond, and mix well. Alternatively, spritz yourself with a sexy body spray. To make this, add about 6–8 drops of your favorite oil blend to a small spray bottle of simple flower water such as rose or orange. Spritz this all over your body for a beautifully fragrant treat.

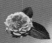

45 Pumpkin and lavender

If you're used to spending a king's ransom on expensive perfumes and colognes, you're in for a surprise. An intriguing research study has discovered that the most effective smell you can use to seduce your man is a combination of pumpkin pie and lavender. As for women, the results show that they respond most erotically to a mixture of licorice and lavender. The tests proved that these specific aromas have a measurable physiological effect, in that they actually increase blood flow to the genitals and boost sexual desire.

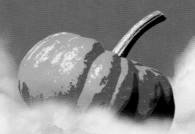

46 Heaps of love

Make a sensual pot pourri for a subliminal aphrodisiac effect, using flowers, herbs, nuts, kernels, cones, wood, and leaves. Choose ingredients that are renowned for their libido-boosting properties. For example: mix dried rose petals, cloves, and cardamom pods, and combine with other dried flowers, dried pods and nuts, and woody pine cones suffused with a few drops of jasmine, ylang-ylang, and neroli essential oils. Arrange in bowls and pots around the room.

47 Kiss, kiss

According to Coco Chanel, you should wear perfume where you want to be kissed. So, if you want to drive your lover wild with your favorite, intoxicating scent, place a few drops on your chosen spot—it may be on your neck; on the nape of your neck; behind your ears; between your breasts; on the inside of your wrists; or behind your knees. Don't use too much scent though—just enough to give off a subtle, delicious aroma that smells good enough to kiss.

48 A hint of musk

If you want to leave your skin smelling deliciously sexy, use musk-scented bath oils, soaps, and body lotions. Or wear a sultry, musky fragrance for a romantic evening with your lover. Musk is one of the most sensuous of smells, because its aroma most closely mimics the scent of human pheromones. There's just one reservation, though: be kind to animals and don't use musk that is derived from wild creatures (e.g., ambergris from the sperm whale or civet from the civet cat). Instead, you should look out for one of the many available synthetic versions or those made from plant sources.

49 Scented hair

Beautiful, shiny, healthy hair is always very alluring. But, apart from ensuring that it looks good, you can make your hair even more enticing by making it smell great as well. Spritz your hair with an aromatic mist to give it a really delicious scent. Make the mist by adding 3–5 drops of essential oil (diluted with a base oil) to a purse-size spray bottle of distilled water. The best oils to use on the hair include: neroli, sandalwood, rose, jasmine, and vanilla. Keep the spray bottle with you and use it to refresh your hair throughout the day.

50 Bed of roses

Suffuse your bedroom with the intoxicating scent of roses. The smell of roses has long been regarded as a natural aphrodisiac. Place freshly cut roses in vases around the room and transform your bedroom into a haven of love. And, while you're at it, sprinkle your bed with fresh rose petals. This is a romantic tradition that has been used for centuries. The Romans used to scatter rose petals at their banquets—not just for the beautiful aroma, but also to promote an erotic mood. For an even more potent effect, add a few drops of rose oil to an oil burner.

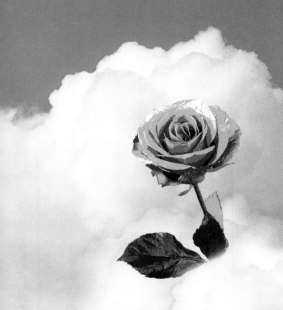

51 Sweet lips

Men simply can't resist a luscious pout. Research shows that women with large, sensual mouths are perceived to be more sexually alluring than those with skinny lips. So, if you want to make yourself instantly more irresistible, draw attention to your kiss appeal with a flattering lipstick or gloss. For an added aphrodisiac effect, use a scented lip color, impregnated with an arousing fragrance. For example, choose a vanilla, strawberry, or rose-scented lip gloss. Or try a lipstick infused with the faintest aroma of chocolate.

52 Foodie scents

Get your partner into an amorous mood by using the delicious scent of food. It's now known that even inhaling the smell of certain foods has a direct aphrodisiac effect. The best foods to try on men include: freshly baked pumpkin pie, cinnamon buns, licorice, and roast meat. Their scents have been shown to raise sexual responsiveness in some men by up to 40 percent. The aromas of other foods such as strawberries, chocolate, vanilla, and peppermint are arousing to both sexes.

53 Body scent

Are you spending a fortune on expensive perfumes to enhance your sex appeal? You don't really need them. One of the most potent aphrodisiac scents is the smell of fresh sweat, so you can turn your lover on with your natural body scent. Legend has it that Napoleon often asked Josephine not to wash for days at a time, because he found the scent of her body so intoxicating. Sweat contains natural chemical scents called pheromones. These act as sexual stimulants, and have a strongly arousing effect on potential lovers. So, the more attracted you are to someone physically, the more you'll love the way he or she smells.

54 Love is in the air

Transform the air around you into a come-hither, sensuous zone by burning incense sticks—especially in the bedroom. Experiment until you find a scent that really suits you: sultry aphrodisiac incenses include patchouli, which has an earthy, musky appeal; sandalwood, for a subtly sensual aroma that helps to stimulate the physical senses; ylang-ylang, for a heavy aphrodisiac effect; jasmine, for a light, loving mood; and frankincense, to calm and soothe. Don't overdo it, though—the effect shouldn't be overwhelming, and don't mix different aromas. It's best to stick to one main scent.

55 Subtly scented

You don't always want an overpowering scent in the air—just a subtle, aphrodisiac aroma. You can achieve this very simply by adding 5–10 drops of essential oils to a bowl of hot water.

Choose from a selection of amorous scents such as ylang-ylang, neroli, sandalwood, jasmine, rose, or cinnamon. (You can combine 2 or 3 oils for a more complex effect.) Leave the bowl uncovered. Another easy way to lightly scent a room is to put a drop of aromatic oil on a light bulb, and then turn it on. Don't drop oil directly onto a hot bulb, however.

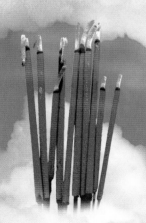

56 Scented undies

Delight your partner by wearing sexily-scented underwear. But first, you need to make a seductive concoction of essential oils. Mix 2 drops of jasmine, and 2 drops of ylang-ylang, with 1 drop of neroli or lime. Dab this onto a cotton wool ball, and rub it over a sheet of wallpaper that you've cut to fit your underwear drawer. Alternatively, just scatter the cotton wool balls inside the drawer. This will keep your underwear beautifully fragrant. Men can use masculine, woody oils such as sandalwood and vetiver.

57 Scented sheets

Make being in bed with your lover an even more erotic experience by scenting the bed linen with libido-boosting scents. The easiest way to do this is to add a few drops of essential oils (e.g., rose, ylang-ylang, or jasmine) to a cotton wool bud, and place it under the pillow covers and bed linen. Or you could place small muslin bags, filled with fresh flowers, spices, and herbs under the pillows. Another aromatic tip is to add some rose water to the final rinse, when you wash your bed linen. And dry yourselves on clean bath towels sprinkled with a few drops of essential oil.

58 Clothes swap

Will you be spending time apart from your lover—for a few days, weeks, even months? If so, you'll miss out on all the invisible but powerful areas of intimacy that affect you subliminally. One of these is the familiar smell of your lover's body. When you're separated, a good way of keeping close is to wear each other's clothes. Choose items that you have worn already and are imbued with the scent of your own natural aroma. Wearing your lover's clothes will act as a sensual reminder and help you to feel close together, even when you are far apart.

59 Bathe your senses

The scent of essential oils acts upon the limbic part of the brain (the part to do with emotions). Different oils will affect you mentally and emotionally, so why not experiment? Try the effects of adding a few drops of rose, neroli, ginger, ylang-ylang, or sandalwood to your bath. Or, make the following sensuous blend:

Ylang-Ylang 3 drops
Rose 3 drops
Sandalwood 3 drops

Dilute the essential oils in a base oil such as jojoba or apricot—1 drop in 5 ml of base oil. Then add 6–8 drops of the blend to your bath, lie back, and enjoy.

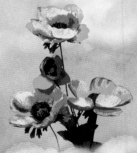

60 Pulse points

Make a special love oil for romantic occasions, and apply it to the pulse points on your temples and wrists:

For her Mix 3 drops ylang-ylang, 2 drops nutmeg, 2 drops vanilla, 2 drops rose, 1 drop jasmine, 1 drop clove, and dilute in an almond oil base.

For him Mix 3 drops sandalwood, 2 drops jasmine, 2 drops ylang-ylang, 1 drop cinnamon, 1 drop clove, and dilute in an almond oil base.

CHAPTER FOUR

seductive mind

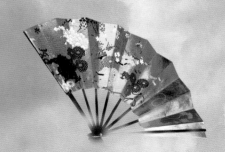

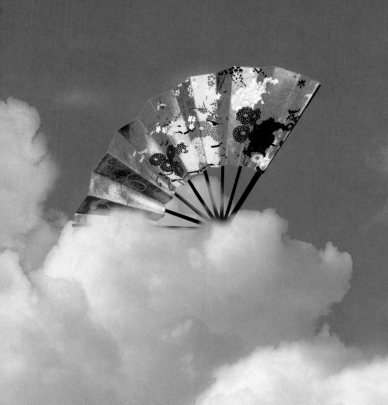

71

61 Pay compliments

Never underestimate the power of compliments—and bombard your lover with admiration. It feels so good to be praised—just think how instantly uplifted you feel. There's a sound physiological reason for this. The feeling of well-being and increased energy is caused by a chemical produced in the brain, which has an effect similar to that of amphetamines. The same chemical is responsible for the emotional high experienced in the early stages of love. Your brain increases production of this every time you are made to feel good about yourself. So, the more approval and attention you receive, the more euphoric you feel.

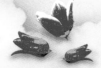

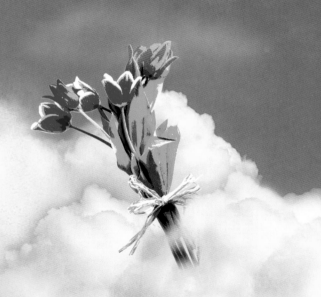

62 Keep a love diary

When you meet your special person, keep a love diary, beginning with the first moment you saw each other. One day this will be a sweet reminder of all those happy times you spent together. Update it as often as you have time—ideally, once a week, but at least once a month. Write down all the things you do together and how you feel. Make a note of important occasions—such as your first kiss, first vacation together, even the first time you have a quarrel. Illustrate your diary with tickets, postcards, love notes, and other precious keepsakes.

63 Make a love album

Gather together the happiest photographs of you and your love, and paste them into a special little album. You must be very selective, though. Choose shots that really capture your most loving, joyful moments—at parties, weddings, at the beach, on a country walk, kissing and hugging each other, or just strolling hand in hand. Write the date and a small caption beside each. Whenever you're in danger of taking each other for granted, get out your album and browse through it together. All the happy vibes will bring back those loving feelings.

64 Clear your mind

If your mind's frazzled, it's difficult to get in the mood for sex.
Tension is a real passion killer—you need to unwind and relax
first, then you'll feel more interested in making love. Try this
simple yoga relaxation breathing technique to reduce your stress
levels. Do it every day for 5–10 minutes.

- Gently pinch your nostrils with your right hand.
- Close your left nostril with your middle and index fingers.
- Inhale slowly and deeply through your right nostril—feel the
  breath right down in your diaphragm. Hold your breath for
  at least 5 seconds.
- Unblock your left nostril. Then block your right nostril with
  your thumb.
- Exhale through your left nostril (while keeping your right
  nostril closed).
- Repeat 10 times. Breathing through alternate nostrils is a very
  effective way to induce feelings of calmness.

65 Get balanced

Here are two simple exercises to get you in the mood for love.

Center yourself Place your left hand a couple of inches below your navel, and cover it with your right hand. Breathe deeply and concentrate on this area for a few minutes until you feel calm.

Balance emotion Sit cross-legged and breathe deeply. Focus on your heart area and see yourself drawing out negative emotions such as anger and anxiety.

66 Read a love poem

Keep a book of love poems by the bed and get into the habit of reading them out loud to each other. This is such a simple thing to do, yet it can really make you both feel intimately connected. Choose favorite poems that you both love. Or, if you prefer, invest in a CD of love poetry. That way, all you have to do is flick on a switch, lie back, listen, and see where the mood takes you.

67 Relax for love

Did you know that about 70 percent of sex problems—including impotence, frigidity, and loss of desire—occur for purely psychological reasons? It's hardly surprising. For great sex, you need to be mentally relaxed, yet physically aroused. Easier said than done if you're feeling stressed, anxious, or worried. This is because negative emotions can leave you feeling hyped up mentally, but physically too depleted to want to do anything— let alone make love. Learn to relax by using strategies such as exercise, massage, meditation, and other relaxation techniques, to transform your sex life.

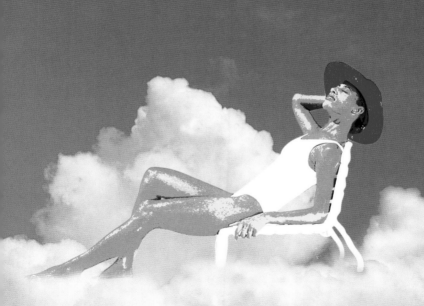

68 A passion anchor

Here's a trick from NLP (neurolinguistic programming) to help keep the passion alive in your relationship. Find a quiet spot and let yourself feel totally relaxed. Close your eyes and think of a situation when you felt really passionate about your partner. Picture it vividly and remember exactly how you felt at the time. As you recall the feeling, press your thumb and forefinger together firmly for a few minutes, to lock those emotions in. This is called making an anchor. Next time you want to get into a passionate frame of mind, simply press your thumb and forefinger together.

69 Love meditation

Use the following meditation to enhance lovemaking:

- Find a quiet place where you can sit comfortably. Close your eyes. Breathe slowly and deeply.
- Imagine a shaft of pure, white light at the crown of your head.

- Direct this shaft of light energy to your heart area.
- Think of your partner and send out total, unconditional, love.
- Feel the love radiating from your heart area and meditate on the words: "I love you with all my heart." Do this for as long as you want.

70 Love visualization

Perhaps you've just had a quarrel, or you and your partner just aren't getting along well any more. When this happens, make a list of ten things that initially attracted you. Was it your lover's voice? smile? eyes? hands? small gestures? Write them all down, then use the following visualization to revive your passion.

- Close your eyes, relax, and think of your partner.
- Choose five points from your list and focus on each one for a minute or so.
- Do this every day for a week to revive those tender feelings.

71 Write love letters

What with e-mail and mobile phones, the art of writing love letters has become redundant. Yet, there's nothing so romantic as receiving an envelope through the post, and finding a passionate note from your lover inside. Try it and see how much pleasure this can bring. It's a good way to keep romantic feelings alive— even if you only write to each other every few months. Save your love letters and keep them in a bundle tied with a red ribbon. Then you can take a quiet moment and read these timeless words to remind yourself how much you are loved.

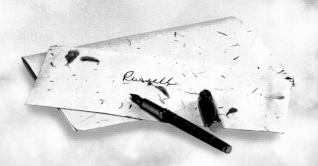

72 Silent seduction

It's often said that sex is mostly in the mind. This is even truer than you think. With practice, you can use your powers of imagination and visualization to transmit erotic passion without moving so much as a whisker. If you find someone deeply attractive, stay calm. Then, quietly and vividly, visualize yourself touching, stroking, and kissing that person, until you're flooded with intense desire. You needn't say a word; your eyes and "vibes" will speak for you. Desire is contagious—and, provided you're both on the same wavelength, your message will be completely understood.

73 Sexual confidence

If shyness is affecting your sex life, you could improve your self-confidence by using self-hypnosis. Do some research first—take a trip to your library or bookstore and look up a reputable course. Providing you learn the correct techniques, you'll be able to go into a trance and communicate positive autosuggestions to yourself. You'll be able to see yourself in a new way; remember, your thoughts radiate out from you and are mirrored back to you by other people. So, when you feel good about yourself, so will others.

74 Seven love checks

Take seven pieces of paper and write something loving about your partner on each. For instance, you may adore the way she or he smiles, cheers you up when you're down, and never fails to surprise you when you least expect it. Get your partner to do the same for you. Shuffle the papers and place them in a box. Pick out a paper each morning and focus on that message for a few minutes before you start your day. This will keep your love alive and remind you how lucky you are to be together.

75 Body image

A lot of problems to do with sex often boil down to how you feel about yourself. For example, you may not feel comfortable about your body; you may feel too fat or too thin. So, here are some tips to improve your body image. Make a list of at least 20 aspects of your body that you value and appreciate—e.g., "I have long legs, beautiful hair, soft skin, lovely eyes, a pretty neck," etc. Then, every day, focus on a chosen part of your body and give it a treat. For example, on your "leg day," have a leg massage, moisturize your legs, and go for a walk. The more you take care of your body, the better you look and feel about yourself.

76 Make eye contact

Remember when you first met? You couldn't stop looking into each other's eyes. According to psychologists, intense eye contact heightens attraction and promotes a deep attachment. It may also be the reason why so many movie stars fall in love with each other while filming—they're in situations where they have to make eye contact all day. If you've been together a while, and want to re-kindle that initial flush of passion, practice gazing into each other's eyes.

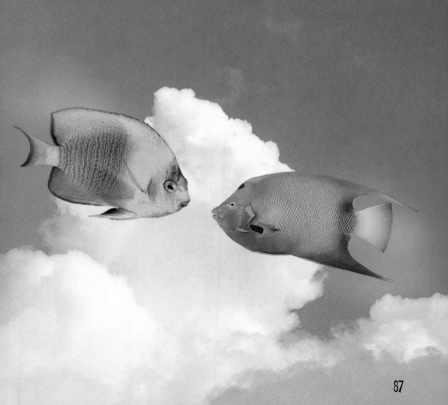

87

77 Put him in the mood for love

Here are some simple ways to put your man in a good mood and ready for love:

- Make him his favorite food.
- Ask him to teach you something that shows his expertise.
- Master the rules of his favorite sport.
- Show an interest in his work.
- Compliment him—men love being praised.

78 Put her in the mood for love

If you want to seduce her, you'll need to make her happy. Here are some tips:

- Flatter her shamelessly. No woman can resist it, but avoid being smarmy.
- Really listen to what she's saying.
- Ask questions about how she feels.

- Tell her that you love the way you can really talk to her.
- Tell her that she drives you wild with desire.

79 Communicate

Good communication is the key to a happy love life. Here are some ways to make sure you and your partner are doing that:

- Smile. It makes you more approachable and your partner will find it hard to resist a smile, even when you are both angry.
- Be a good listener. People clam up when they feel they aren't being heard.
- Mirror your partner's actions. This will subconsciously make him or her want to relax and open up, because he or she feels you're on the same wavelength.
- Listen to your lover's cues. Are they auditory ("I hear what you mean"), visual ("I see what you mean"), or kinesthetic (touchy, feely)? Try to communicate back in the same way.

80 Kiss and make up

Had an argument? Here are some ways to kiss and make up:

- Try to look at the funny side.
- Go off for a few minutes and breathe calmly and deeply. This will help you to feel less tense.
- Send good thoughts to your partner. This will make you feel more warmly affectionate and the "vibes" will convey your peaceful intentions.
- Suggest you give your lover a relaxing massage—and see where it takes you!

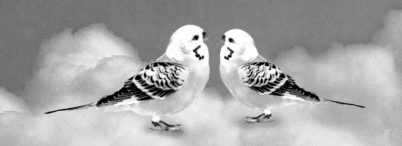

seductive space

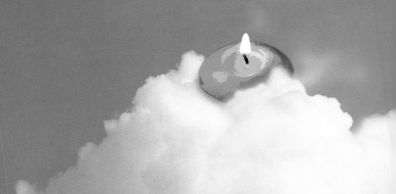

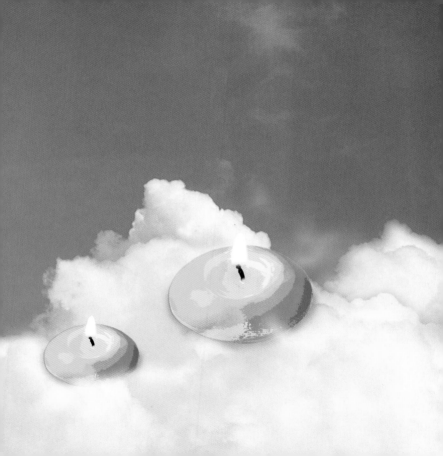

81 A comfortable bed

Is your bed the perfect place for romance? Think about it. You may be accustomed to your familiar old mattress, but it might be a real turn-off for your lover. Your bed should be an oasis of comfort and sensual pleasure—but if it's not, then it might be a good idea to purchase a new one. You can also make your bed alluring and welcoming by choosing pretty bed linen, soft pillows, and piles of snuggly cushions. For a touch of fragrance, place scented sachets inside cushion covers or under your pillow.

82 Loving reflections

Feng shui experts forbid placing a mirror in front of your bed because this will hinder your forward progress. However, this doesn't mean that you can't enjoy the effect of using them elsewhere in your bedroom and the rest of the house. Mirrors are a wonderful way of beaming extra light to your space, and cleverly sited, can also reflect pretty views of the outside world. You can gaze at the vista together while lying in bed; also, of course, there's nothing quite as romantic as looking into a mirror as you kiss and hold each other..

83 Set the scene

It doesn't take much to transform the atmosphere of your bedroom so that it becomes a haven of peace and serenity. Clear away untidy piles of clothes and clutter, switch off any harsh overhead lights, and use bedside lamps instead. You could also use candles to create a romantic mood—the warm glow has a relaxing, feel-good effect and helps to get you and your lover in the mood for love. Candles are available in pretty colors and delicious scents—so make a collection of your favorites and use them to suit your emotions. Purple, pink, and lavender all evoke romance, but to inspire intense feelings of passion, choose red.

84 Two by two

The Chinese believe that if you want to stay together, you should always arrange decorative accessories in pairs, especially in the bedroom. For example, you should display two red candles, two framed photographs, two matching paintings, or two mandarin ducks. Mandarin ducks are particularly favored to bring luck in love—ideally, they should be made of rose quartz and tied together with a red ribbon. If you have twin beds, these should also be identically accessorized—each perfectly matched up with a lamp and table at the side.

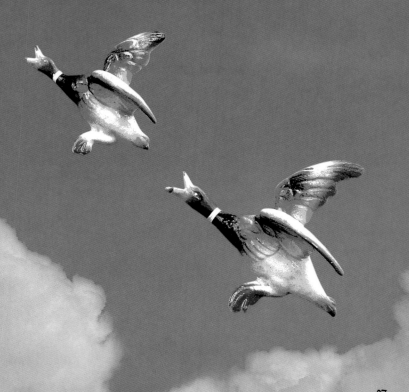

85 Paint it red

Want a red hot sex life? Then paint your bedroom red, if you dare. Every color gives off a unique vibration that affects your body on a physiological level. Red is the hottest color—and this means it is naturally the most arousing. Just looking at red raises your blood pressure, stimulates your heart, and has an energizing effect. So, if you want more excitement in bed, you will need to see red. You may not want to go to the extreme of painting the entire room, of course. In that case, simply add a splash of red in the form of accessories—try scarlet lampshades, red cushions, or a dramatic red throw.

86 In the pink

To invoke a gentle mood of romance in your home, try adding subtle touches of pink to your surroundings. For instance, you can use pink sheets on your bed, scatter some pink cushions, light groups of pink candles, or you can paint your bedroom walls pink. The effect is immensely soft and soothing. In color therapy, pink is the color of romance—it gives off a warm, loving vibration. It's also a good color to choose if you're single—its vibrational energy helps you to attract love and romance.

87 Crystal clarity

Improve your love life by using crystals in your home. Crystal therapists say that each type of crystal has a specific vibration. Just holding, or being near, a particular crystal can influence the energies of your body. The gentle energy of rose quartz is closely associated with love and romance, and crystal experts say that hanging rose quartz crystals in the bedroom will improve your love life. Other beneficial crystals include: garnet, which works on heart energy; topaz, which helps to disperse anger, depression, and jealousy; and turquoise, which is calming and healing.

88 Seductive sounds

Fill your living space with the right music, and your lover
will be putty in your hands. Music can have a powerful
physiological effect on the body; it's now known that
certain sounds speed up the circulation and heart rate,
and make you feel more aroused. For instance, classical music
closely matches the natural rhythms of the heart and has a
directly stimulating effect. Most of us have our special songs or
melodies that evoke memories of shared love and desire; so,
make sure you discover the sounds that excite your lover. Then
use the amazing power of the music to work its erotic magic.

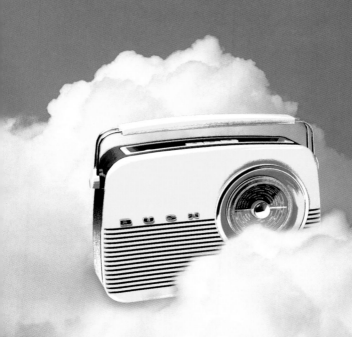

89 Plant a red peony

The Chinese believe that a red peony symbolizes harmony, love, and a happy marriage. The scent is considered to have great aphrodisiac properties; moreover, its deep red shade represents blood, a powerful color for love. That's why this beautiful flower is always given to a newly married couple at a Chinese wedding, to wish them good luck. You don't have to get married to enhance your love life, however; simply plant a red peony in the southwest area of your garden.

90 Loving pictures

According to oriental wisdom, if you want to maintain a harmonious, vibrant relationship, it's important to surround yourself with positive images of yourself and your partner. This means that you should display only those photographs that show you looking really happy together. Sad, melancholy images are considered to attract a similar kind of energy, whereas your lively, smiling faces will energize your home and reinforce the passions of your love life.

91 Perfect harmony

If you want to improve your love life, bring a serene mood of balance and harmony to your environment by de-cluttering the southwest area of your home. According to the laws of feng shui, the ancient Chinese technique of arranging your living space to enhance positive energy flow, this area is associated with your personal relationships. Untidy piles of objects such as books and magazines impede the free flow of energy. This could cause arguments and conflicts with your partner. So, do a thorough spring cleaning to introduce a sense order and clarity. Then revitalize the area by making it brighter and lighter—try changing the lighting or even burning some candles.

92 Fresh Flowers

You can make your surroundings more romantic with pots of gorgeous fresh flowers. Choose blooms that are most associated with love and passion. In Victorian times, flowers were exchanged almost like a secret code—each flower had a meaning, which the recipient would understand. Here are just a few examples:

Red and pink roses for true love

White roses for eternal love

Red and white roses for unity

Bluebells for fidelity

Orchids for everlasting love

Sunflowers for loyalty

Tulips for beautiful eyes

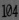

93 Light a fire

What could be more romantic than an
open fire? There's something hypnotic
about the sight of leaping flames that helps
to get you and your partner in a relaxed mood for
loving. If your home doesn't have a fireplace, then seek out
a place that does. Take a romantic break together at an old-
fashioned country hotel or a mountain chalet. Here you can
spend a few days hidden away, just the two of you, enjoying the
country air, some good food and wine, and lots of magic
moments in the firelight.

94 Fabulous fur

There's nothing quite like the soft, silky texture of fur on bare skin to get your senses aroused. So why not try using fur in your living space—especially during the winter months? Nowadays, you can buy the most exquisite "faux fur" soft furnishing items such as rugs, throws, and cushions—so you can be kind to animals, while enjoying a touch of unashamed luxury at the same time. When it's cold and dark outside, enjoy relaxing with your lover on a cozy fur rug in front of an open fire, or snuggle under a sumptuous fur throw on your bed. It's a little bit of heaven.

95 Watch the fish

You and your partner need to be completely relaxed to be in the right mood for happy sex—and that can be hard to attain in today's busy world. However, there are various ways to induce this desirable state of calm. One strategy is to invest in a tank of tropical fish—especially now that modern designers have invented such ingenious ways of integrating these into domestic interiors. A subtly lit tank with exquisite fish gently flitting through the watery depths induces a zen-like state of peace in the room; so, wind down together as you watch the fish, then relax in each other's arms, and see where the moment takes you.

96 Indoor jungle

It's now widely agreed that plants have a positively beneficial effect on your living space. Your home may be affected by all kinds of hidden environmental influences such as chemicals used in cleaning materials. Consequently, it's a good idea to use plants on a generous scale, as they are superb at filtering out toxins from the air. Your plants will not only look beautiful and luxuriant, they will thrive better when they are arranged in groups. They keep each other healthy, while improving the air you breathe.

97 Bathroom haven

If you want to make the most of your living space, transform your bathroom into a sensuous pleasure zone. Make sure that it's clean, softly lit, comfortably warm, with heated towel rails, and equipped with plenty of fluffy towels. Arrange pretty bottles of bath oils on the shelves, choose deliciously scented soaps, and natural bath sponges. And display a few exquisite objects such as a perfect shell or stone. You can also burn scented candles and essential oils such as jasmine and ylang-ylang to enjoy as you bask in your bath. Sip a glass of champagne as you luxuriate, and don't forget to invite your lover in to share the pleasure.

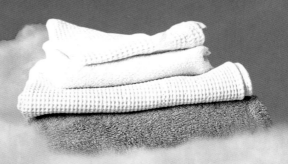

98 Kitchen seduction

Your kitchen may be supremely cool and modern or sweetly old fashioned and traditional—the style doesn't matter at all. It's what you cook that makes your lover go weak at the knees. Studies have shown that the aromas of certain foods can trigger intensely pleasurable sensations in the brain, producing a euphoric, feel-good state. So, if you want to get your lover in a wonderfully loving mood, prepare food that not only tastes delicious, but smells enticing as well. Fill the air with the scent of cinnamon or the aroma of pumpkin pie; in no time at all, you'll be wafted out of the kitchen and into the bedroom.

99 Perfect peace

When the rest of your living space is busy, noisy, and full of activity, it's important to try to keep at least one area completely private, calm, and comfortable. Your bedroom is probably the easiest place to turn into a hideaway for you and your partner. It should be free from the sounds of telephones, television, and anything else that can disturb your peace. Use the most soothing colors and lighting here, fill the space with flowers and plants, and play gentle, relaxing music. This means that no matter what else is going on in your lives, you'll always have a special haven where you can retreat together.

100 Colors in your space

The colors of your surroundings will have a direct effect on your emotions and sense of well-being, so choose your decorating shades with care. The better your mood, the easier it is to be loving—that's why gentle shades such as soft yellow, pink, cream, and terracotta are so popular. They are all feel-good colors. Peach and apricot tones will also make you and your lover feel noticeably relaxed, and green is beautifully calming.

acknowledgments

Cover photograph © Anup Shah/Nature Picture Library